Encore
Wellness & Weight Loss

A Balanced and Inspired Toolkit for Maintaining Weight Loss Success

Donald R. Henderson, M. D., MPH
Monica L. Holt

ISBN-10: 0-692-61215-7
ISBN-13: 978-0-692-61215-6

We dedicate this book to all Encore members and to those who have struggled to maintain a healthy weight.

We would also like to thank our Encore staff for their years of dedication to this mission.

TABLE OF CONTENTS

ENCORE MISSION STATEMENT

Encore Wellness & Weight Loss is a healthcare company based in Southern California that has created a movement to encourage individuals to take control of improving their health. Along with coaching and support services, we give our members the tools needed to make lasting lifestyle changes.

Diet and nutrition is our central focus. We recognize that overall health can be improved by managing weight. Many diseases and disorders are worsened by improper nutrition and the lack of weight management. We strive to be a committed health partner.

Our protocols for lifestyle modification are based upon established medical principles. Encore has revolutionized the way members define weight loss, wellness and a healthy lifestyle. By interconnecting core values with rituals that include balanced nutrition and fitness, Encore delivers sustainable weight loss and nutrition solutions that lead to a healthier, more balanced life.

We believe that healthcare should be supervised and delivered by licensed physicians and health practitioners in a compassionate and confidential environment. We remain committed to delivering quality treatment and support services to enhance overall health.

We encourage you to use Encore's Prescription to Live your Best Life and Live Longer.

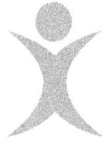

WELCOME TO THE ENCORE WAY OF LIVING!

YOUR PRESCRIPTION FOR LIVING A LONGER, HEALTHIER LIFE

Losing weight can be a challenge for some. Here are the numbers to prove it.

Current statistics indicate that the obesity rate for African-Americans is 47.8%, for Latino Americans, 42.5% and for Caucasian Americans, the obesity rate is 32.6%.

Advertisers promote the consumption of inexpensive, unhealthy fast food. This worldwide trend has led to the consumption of foods that encourage weight gain and obesity. To change the trend and have a positive impact on your health from this day forward, you must decide to consume food that promotes good nutrition and provides you with the energy you need to be productive.

Every week, we make more than one hundred food choices. To ensure that you know the importance of making the best food choice, Encore has developed your prescription for a longer and healthier life.

This Encore prescription contains guidelines and rituals that will help you establish a new relationship with food. You will receive a roadmap that guides you to the right food choices. When you make good nutrition a priority, and when you incorporate healthy rituals into your day, you will notice that you're reducing calories, spending less on food and feeling better than ever!

As you move through each stage of the Encore program, you will see how important it is to adopt healthy daily rituals. Just as brushing your teeth is a ritual you established at an early age, the healthy choices you make today regarding food and exercise will become habits or rituals that will improve your quality of life.

We are sharing this program to serve as your roadmap to a new way of life. The Encore Prescription can be a reference tool that will help you stay on track to obtain and maintain a healthy weight for a lifetime.

We encourage you to become an Encore member and obtain the resources needed to educate your family on the best ways to maintain optimal health.

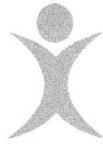

TIP

Go to www.encoreweightloss.com to learn more about our coaching tools and programs that promote good health and sustainable results.

THE ENCORE PRESCRIPTION FOR WEIGHT LOSS
THREE KEY STAGES:

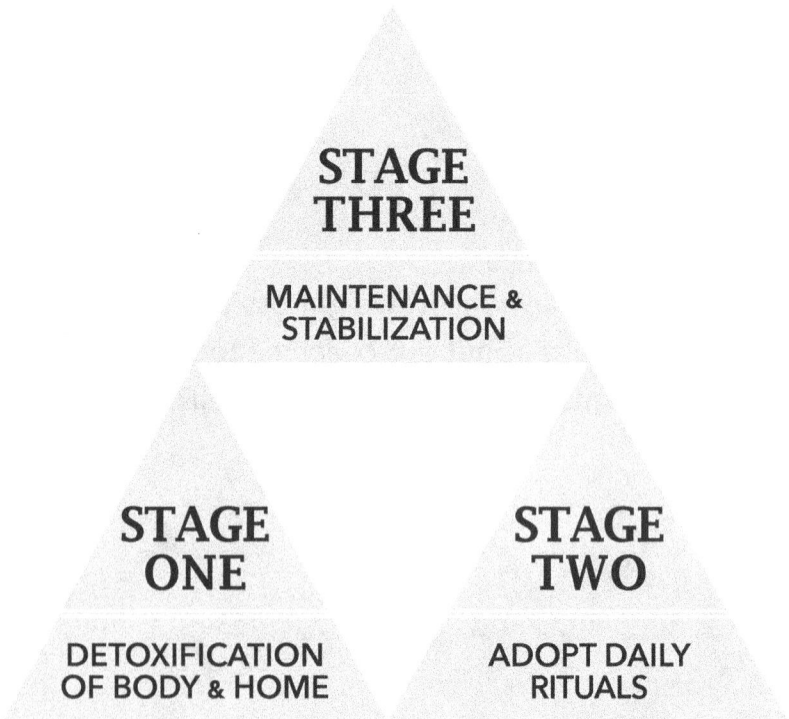

STAGE THREE

MAINTENANCE & STABILIZATION

STAGE ONE

DETOXIFICATION OF BODY & HOME

STAGE TWO

ADOPT DAILY RITUALS

THE ENCORE DIFFERENCE: OUR APPROACH TO FORMING NEW HABITS FOR A NEW LIFE

Encore Wellness & Weight Loss is a medically-supervised weight loss program that shows you how to hit the reset button. We proactively guide you toward total wellness and use a variety of tools to accomplish this.

The Encore prescription is available in our medical offices in Southern California as well as through our Encore Associates' medical offices nationwide. Encore's virtual office is accessible through our website's personalized patient portal. We offer remote healthcare monitoring that includes personalized biometric data evaluation. We can track weight, heart rate, blood pressure, activity levels and other vital statistics.

A key component of wellness is weight loss. We believe that maintaining a healthy weight will help determine how your body responds to other health risks. In the medical office, Encore's new member assessment begins with a complete physical examination, body measurements and a full spectrum of laboratory tests. If medically indicated, we suggest advanced testing and coordinate the findings with your personal physician. If you visit our virtual office, we recommend including your physician in the process to maximize your results and manage any health concerns you may have.

Based upon the initial assessment, Encore healthcare providers prescribe a program that may include a combination of balanced nutrition meal plans, vitamins, supplements and journaling. Members also receive a set of rituals that help establish new dietary habits. The initial 4-6 week program will include comprehensive weight loss management and follow-up care. Producing significant, life-changing results is our primary objective. This objective is attainable by changing perceptions of and the relationship with food.

- We believe the use of Encore's healthy rituals will lead to improved nutrition and lead to a longer, healthier life.

- We believe the linking of healthy rituals and gratitude journaling provides the power needed to make positive and sustainable life changes.

We work with members to select the most appropriate meal plan, supplements and fitness program that best work to achieve total wellness and sustainable weight loss. Our goal is to provide the tools to maintain a practical health regimen for a lifetime.

WEIGH IN ON THE FACTS

Being overweight and obese are associated with an increased risk for diabetes, heart disease, stroke, cancer, arthritis, infertility, sleep apnea, asthma and depression.

At the current rate of weight gain, by the year 2030 more than two-thirds of Americans will be obese. Obese patients spend $1,500 more per year on healthcare, compared to patients of average weight.

The number of overweight and obese people around the world has steadily increased.

- Today more than fifty percent (50%) of American adults are overweight and more than 17% of children are obese.

- At the current rate of growth, medical complications from obesity could bankrupt the healthcare system. Poor diet and lifestyle cause eighty percent (80%) of chronic disease and currently cost the U.S. over $500 billion annually.

- Years ago, the average weight gain after age 30 was 1/2 pound per year; today the average adult gains 1-2 pounds per year.

- Most overweight people think they are in good health, yet they take an average of 3 or more medications for chronic medical conditions.

Unfortunately, the food industry is a direct contributor to obesity. It constantly pushes nutrition myths that cause us to make the wrong food choices.

The quality of your lifestyle and personal health status can be determined by the use of seven important variables. If you are able to control these seven medical variables, you will have found the fountain of youth. Adoption of these seven medical variables can help you live longer and require fewer medical treatments.

TIP

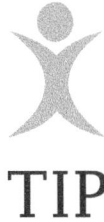

SEVEN MEDICAL VARIABLES TO IMPROVE QUALITY OF LIFE

1. Consume a diet low in fat, moderate in quality protein and high in fruits, vegetables and grain. Focus on eating a plant-based diet

2. Be consistent with daily physical activity

3. If you're a smoker, STOP

4. Maintain a sense of community and spiritual connection

5. Monitor blood pressure

6. Monitor blood sugar

7. Monitor cholesterol

If you're committed to making a change, let's get started!

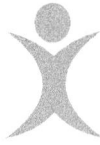

STAGE ONE
DETOXIFICATION OF BODY & HOME

To jump-start weight loss and to increase energy levels, the Encore prescription begins with a total body cleanse.

There are many ways to cleanse your body. The important point is that you need to release current or past waste. This simple act of cleansing your colon will make you feel better. Ridding your body of waste provides a template for improved body physiology. Think of your body as an engine. Buying the wrong kind of gasoline may lead to engine knocks and incomplete combustion. Our cells burn food energy just as your car engine burns gasoline. When you combine ineffective and improperly balanced food into your diet, the resulting ineffective physiologic combustion will lead to sludge buildup in the arteries of your heart, kidney, brain, liver and other vital organs.

WHY DEEP CLEANSE?

- STIMULATES FAT BURNING
  The reduction of calories on cleanse days
  stimulates the body's fat-burning furnaces
  while suppressing fat synthesis and
  storage.

- TRIGGERS DETOXIFICATION
  The absence of food on cleanse days gives
  the digestion processes a break, allowing
  the liver to do its job of detoxifying the
  body. Deep cleansing also stimulates the
  release of stored fat-soluble toxins.

- REDUCES OXIDATIVE STRESS & INFLAMMATION
  As fat cells shrink, they release fewer
  signaling molecules that cause oxidative
  stress and inflammation. Reducing total
  body fat also helps improve antioxidant
  status in the body. Oxidative stress, in
  particular, plays a large role in bioactivity
  related to aging. As you lower the
  oxidative stress levels, you slow the aging
  process.

How the Body's Detox System Works

The body has its own extraordinary internal detoxification system. Here's a brief look at three critical organs involved:

- THE LIVER: Your first line of defense against toxins is your liver. The liver acts like a filter in preventing toxic substances contained in foods and the environment from passing into your body's systems.

- THE INTESTINE: This organ has bacteria that produce both healthy and unhealthy chemicals. You want to keep your colon flowing regularly. The colon's main role is to flush out harmful toxins before they can cause inflammation.

- THE KIDNEYS: The kidneys are constantly filtering your blood to get rid of toxins.

Purging and the associated modified fasting helps your body to detoxify and reset the microscopic environment of your intestinal tract. Your intestines contain as many bacteria, viruses and microbes as the total number of cells in the rest of your body. Many of these intestinal microbes can be directly related to weight gain. A health small bowel microbe population is essential to digestive health.

The Encore system of body purge promotes the establishment of a new, more balanced gastrointestinal environment that is more conducive to weight loss and weight loss maintenance.

THE ENCORE PROTOCOL • 2-DAY DEEP CLEANSE

- Drink one-half to one gallon of water throughout the day. Consult your healthcare provider to determine the safety of water intake.

- Mid-morning snack: eat one cup of strawberries, blueberries or grapefruit pieces.

- Take two large tablespoons of polyethylene glycol laxative in a large glass of water - morning, afternoon and evening.

- Be mindful of your diet. Eat foods low in fat and sugar.

- Practice portion control.

- Reduce the pace of your eating. Chew slowly.

- If needed, use an Encore recommended cleanse product or laxative preparation.

BREAKFAST

We recommend a low-calorie cereal or oatmeal with low-fat milk and fruit. A mid-morning snack of berries is suggested to curb hunger and accelerate the cleansing process.

LUNCH

Be mindful of your total caloric intake. Choose foods that provide pleasure but purposefully limit the volume you eat.

- Mid-afternoon snack: enjoy 1 large cup of one of the following vegetables steamed, grilled (without oil) or gently boiled:

  - Spinach
  - Chard
  - Tomatoes
  - Celery
  - Fennel
  - Cucumbers
  - Asparagus or
  - Cabbage
  - Drink More Water throughout the Day!

DINNER

- Repeat the fruits and vegetables from earlier today, add 1 cup of yogurt.
- Consume a low-fat dinner of your choice.
- Record the total calories you've eaten for the day.
- Record your number of bowel movements.
- Relax at the end of the day with a cup of chamomile tea.

On Cleanse days, only participate in light to moderate workouts. Consider yoga, stretching or walking. You may not begin to experience bowel movements until the second day of the cleanse. If you experience nausea or any symptoms that alarm you, consult your healthcare provider.

In some ways, cleansing represents a modified fasting state. Fasting allows your body to burn fat as stored energy. Fasting may slow aging. With moderate fasting our cells produce fewer free radicals that age our bodies. The reduction of free radicals allow our cells to last longer and function more efficiently.

SET THE STAGE FOR SUCCESS AT HOME

As you prepare the mind and body for a transforming experience, you must also clear your home. Unhealthy foods and snacks work against your weight loss goals.

- Acknowledge your personal trigger foods and avoid them.

- Remove from your environment foods that tempt you. Then it will be much easier to follow your Encore Meal Plan.

Search your freezer, pantry and cabinets for unhealthy foods and remove them. Focus on removing foods that are processed or high in fat, salt or sugar, yet low in nutritional value. Get rid of the potato chips, cookies candy and other unhealthy foods. Restock your house with plant-based foods. Keep healthy quantities of fresh fruit and nuts on hand. Plan to limit your intake of meats and other processed foods.

Skipping Meals

Skipping meals is not a good idea and doesn't actually produce the results you might expect. Here are a few important nutritional facts to consider:

> ➤ Skipping meals, especially breakfast, can actually lead to weight gain.

> ➤ When you skip meals, you are not giving your body the fuel it needs to properly function.

> ➤ Skipping meals is known to cause low blood sugar and may lead to impulse eating.

> ➤ Skipping meals encourages poor eating habits and cravings for late night poor food choices.

Please refer to the Appendix for food suggestions that can support you throughout the program.

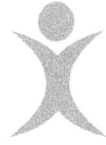

TIP

Spread your total caloric intake throughout the day. Try to make breakfast your most important and largest meal. Your next largest meal should be lunch. At dinner design food choices that do not include large volumes of food. Eat breakfast like a king, lunch like a prince, followed by a small quantity for dinner.

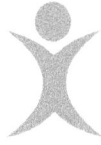

STAGE TWO
THE ENCORE METHOD & EMBRACING DAILY RITUALS

Each year you may eat as many as 1,200 meals. Your food choices most often are not related to careful consideration but are related to reflex and to habits. Developing new habits with food selections require a new focused on dietary rituals. If you follow the Encore dietary rituals for 4 to 6 weeks, your chances of successfully developing new dietary habits will significantly increase.

To be happier and to live longer requires that you focus on those habits that may control 80% of your life.

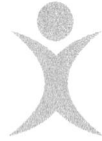

TIP

How to Create Positive Change in Your Life

- 40-80% of our life decisions are based upon habits.

- Rituals are the building blocks of habits.

- The linking of values to daily rituals provide a powerful platform for life change.

Encore programs identify "keystone" nutritional bad habits and provide daily dietary rituals that can help you establish good dietary habits. Habit formation is a complex idea yet a simple process. Encore's set of dietary rituals are easy to understand.

Simplicity is power. Stage Two focuses on the effective combination of values mixed with new dietary rituals and caloric restriction.

After using the Encore method for 45 days, you will see and feel a difference in how your body performs.

WHY DO WE EAT?

The answer should be because we are hungry and because we want to maintain our body's energy throughout the day. In reality, we eat for a variety of other reasons. We eat to socialize with friends. We eat to celebrate special occasions. We eat for comfort. When food becomes a comfort, it can lead to emotional eating. Emotional eating should be recognized as an abnormal eating pattern and can be a major cause of weight gain.

Are you ready to make the change?

- *Readiness for Change*: Do you have the resources and knowledge to successfully make a lasting change?

- *Barriers to Change*: Is there anything that's preventing you from changing?

- *Expect Relapse*: What triggers a return to a former behavior?

The Encore program provides guidelines for changing poor dietary habits. It's important to recognize that changing behavior is not an easy process but can be accomplished with the right tools. At Encore, we prepare you with the correct tools and help get you through the initial resistance to change.

It's Time To Get Mentally Prepared

A way to address mindless emotional eating is to mentally prepare yourself for weight loss.

A Stanford University School of Medicine study suggests that overweight people who learn skills to maintain their weight loss before starting a plan maintained 80-90% of their weight loss after meeting their goals.

By adopting Encore's philosophy and practicing healthy rituals, you will begin to understand why you overeat. You can then develop the tools to defeat overeating, and keeping the weight off will be much easier and less stressful. The key is to learn ways to prevent old habits from taking control of your life. The key is to use the Encore rituals to develop new, healthy habits.

Learning maintenance skills before rather than after starting a weight loss program will increase the likelihood of long-term success.

Whether your goal is to lose weight or to improve your seven (7) Medical Variables outlined above, there is no single solution that works for everyone. You may need to try several different techniques to find the right combination of daily rituals that work for you...and that keep you motivated to succeed.

HEALTHY RITUALS

To increase your chance of weight loss success, start by adopting healthy rituals. These real-world skills can help you prepare for and maintain your weight loss.

Encore rituals are your points of action and must be reinforced daily.

Reinforcing occurs by daily reading of your rituals. Daily ritual reading repetition provides a greater chance for behavior change. Your weight is the most visible part of your overall health. Your blood pressure and cholesterol levels are important but less visible.

A small change in your current weight provides tremendous health benefits. To obtain that benefit you have to develop new habits based upon Encore's rituals. Adopt and read each set of rituals as part of your daily routine. To help you reach your health goals, Encore's rituals demand your attention and must be read each morning and reviewed several times throughout the day. Repetition reinforces your goal and reminds you why you're making this commitment to your health.

This prescription for a longer, happier life provides rituals that are situational. We have touched upon rituals for almost every activity of daily living. However, we encourage you to add your own rituals to personalize the process and increase your chances for success.

Psychological Rituals

- Always be honest with yourself and set attainable goals.

- Say no to second servings, turn down the donut, don't taste the ice cream.

- Enter everything you eat throughout the day into your Encore Daily Journal or a weight loss app.

- Avoid panic eating by planning ahead and having healthy snacks close by.

- Avoid consuming empty calories, including alcoholic beverages and sugary drinks.

- Avoid the Starbucks craze.

- Enjoy the success of being able to say no to things that tempt you.

- Learn to be satisfied with eating less.

- Stay mindful of your presence and your purpose.

- Think about where you are and what your goal is.

Encore rituals can be applied to all aspects of your life. As you define your goals, apply these guidelines for better results:

1. Be specific with your goal.

2. Set realistic goals that can be accomplished.

3. Your goals should allow for flexibility.

When you psychologically sabotage your efforts by setting unrealistic goals, you get discouraged when you cannot accomplish them.

Another useful technique to accomplish large goals is to set a series of short-term goals that gets you closer to your ultimate goal.

Social Rituals

- Surround yourself with inspiring and supportive family, co-workers and friends.

- Remind yourself daily how far you've come on this journey. You've invested time and emotions in your weight loss journey that you can never get back again. Why start over?

- Don't allow your social network to pressure you into eating poorly at outings. What you see everyone else ordering to drink or eat does not have to apply to you.

- Get in the habit of rewarding yourself with something you value other than food.

Begin to recognize the cues that lead to overeating in your weekly routine. When you review your daily food journal, you may find that you overeat while watching TV or when gathering with certain friends. When you change the situation and separate activity from food, you can then successfully manage your health and will see improved results.

DIETARY RITUALS: EATING PATTERNS

- Select smaller food portions. Some cultures stop eating when full, yet Americans eat for volume and not fullness. Create a new fullness set point.

- Eat slower. Your brain takes time to realize that you are full.

- Chew your food at least eight times before swallowing.

- Pause between swallowing and getting the next forkful.

- Put your fork down while chewing.

- Reduce carbohydrates found in sweet desserts and drinks; eat fruit instead.

- Take half forkfuls of food.

- Try to consume an 8-oz glass of water prior to your meal.

- Only drink water with your meal, at least two 8-oz glasses per setting.

- Avoid fried foods, rice, potatoes, pasta, chips and breads.

- Don't eat while driving.

- Don't eat while standing...we tend to eat more.

Each day you must commit yourself to the idea of success and the actions connected to success. If you want to lose weight, then you must take steps toward living Encore's daily dietary rituals. Each morning and at least three times during the day read or recall at least one dietary ritual.

Physical Rituals

- Develop an exercise program that gradually increases your activity level and fits your lifestyle.

- Walk as much as possible.

- Avoid the closest parking space; use this time to add steps to your pedometer.

- Weigh yourself every day around the same time, under the same circumstances.

- Each morning empty your bladder and your bowel, then weigh yourself prior to dressing.

- Always use the same scale.

- Keep track of your weight at home. Always provide that weight to your healthcare providers.

- Create new routines around your new schedule that reinforce and support your new goals.

- Keep 100-calorie snack packs (crackers, yogurts, fruit, etc.) in your car, office, briefcase or purse.

- Avoid all soft drinks (diet and regular), fruit juices and processed smoothies.

You will not be able to exercise your way to weight loss. Physical activity does play an important role. When combined with dietary changes, increased physical activity provides a key ingredient toward long-term success.

Gratitude Journaling

Studies have shown that keeping a Gratitude Journal acts as a natural antidepressant. Gratitude documentation can even increase your level of overall happiness. Gratitude is the greatest of all virtues. Gratitude journaling provides the power needed for making life changes.

Here are 5 ways you can maximize the benefits of Gratitude Journaling:

1) Keep a Daily Gratitude Journal

This is probably the most effective strategy for increasing your level of gratitude. Set aside time each day to record several things that you are grateful for in your life. Choose a consistent time of day when you're able to reflect on things that impact your day and your life.

The important thing is to establish the daily practice of paying attention to gratitude-inspiring events and to write them down. It has been said the act of writing "allows you to see the meaning of events going on around you and create meaning in your own life." For an example of the use of a gratitude journal, see Joan Buchman's article "The Healing Power of Gratitude."

2) USE VISUAL REMINDERS

Two obstacles to being grateful are forgetfulness and lack of awareness. You can counter both obstacles by giving yourself visual cues that trigger thoughts of gratitude. Consider listing your blessings on Post-it notes and placing them where you'll easily see them. Another strategy is to set a reminder on your computer or phone to signal you at random times during the day to pause and count your blessings.

3) HAVE A GRATITUDE PARTNER

Social support encourages healthy behaviors because we often lack the discipline to do things on our own. Just as you may be more likely to exercise if you have an exercise partner, you may be able to maintain the discipline of gratitude journaling if you have a partner to share your lists and discuss the effects of gratitude in your life.

4) MAKE A PUBLIC COMMITMENT

We feel accountable when we make commitments to others. Set weekly goals for yourself and share them with those close to you. The fact that the goal is made publicly to a group increases the likelihood that you will follow through and achieve it.

5) CHANGE YOUR SELF-TALK

We all carry on an inner dialogue with ourselves that is often called "self-talk." When this inner conversation is negative, it can lower our mood and lead to depression. Research has shown that we can change our mood by changing the tone of the things we say to ourselves. Remember, what we think becomes reality, so stay positive!

30-Day Routine of an Encore Program

When you enroll as a member of Encore, you will receive a customized regimen. Below is an example of a typical 4-week program.

Days 1-2: Critical To Your Success

- Weigh yourself at the same time each day after emptying your bladder or bowel, but before dressing. Record your weight in the Encore Journal

- Drink 1/2 to 1 gallon of water throughout the day. Disclose any medical needs for fluid restriction.

- To increase metabolic levels, commit to a minimum of 20-60 minutes of cardio activity three times per week to burn fat and increase energy levels.

- Conduct physical activity in the morning. For maximum results, try to book-end your day with physical activity – 30 minutes in the morning and 30 minutes in the evening.

- Physical activity means walking. Increase your activity as medically permissible.

- Weigh yourself at the same time each day after emptying your bladder or bowel, but before dressing. Record your weight in the Encore Journal.

- Take your daily dietary supplements.

- Drink 1/2 to 1 gallon of water throughout the day.

- Follow your customized meal plan calorie count that has been designed for you.

- Consult with your Encore Weight Loss Coach for tips on food selection, meal preparation and to help you stay motivated!

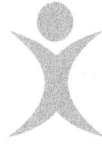

STAGE THREE
ENCORE'S MAINTENANCE PROGRAM, "MAINTAIN FOR LIFE"

You are nearing or have reached your desired weight. The decisions you've made up to this point represent a commitment of time, effort and willpower.

To ensure success you have to pay close attention to the Encore rituals. You have to learn how to eat to live a longer healthier life. The confusion and pressure associated with every day life provides a template for falling off the wagon. Creating new habits by learning new rituals is the most powerful tool at your disposal.

Each day our food choices are impacted by our desires far less than by marketing and governmental regulations. We are driven to eat more of the wrong type of foods. We are bombarded with subliminal messages indicating that we are hungry. We are presented with cheap foods that are high in sugar, salt and fats.

During the first 30 days of your Encore program you will have to learn how to eat differently. To love food and savor the flavors, eat slowly. Chew each bite at least eight times prior to swallowing. Examine the flavor and complexity of the food as you are chewing. Learn the difference between feeling full and feeling stuffed. If you are tuned into that difference, you can easily lose 20 pounds in 30 days.

Your body is like an automobile. You only need so much gas to operate each 24 hour cycle of life. So, don't overstuff your food tank with excess calories. If you do, these calories will turn into fat.

Discontinue all mindless snacking and that includes eating while driving.

The key question to ask yourself: How will you keep the pounds off? Encore understands the difficulty one faces when trying to maintain weight loss success.

To achieve long-term weight loss success, we encourage you to use Encore's weight maintenance program. MAINTAIN FOR LIFE should be employed for a minimum of 8 weeks after you've reached your desired weight. This will help you reinforce and establish new behaviors and rituals that you can continue for a lifetime.

It's time to hit the health-reset button and learn how to support and reinforce the healthy new you!

What Is Weight Loss Success?

To obtain long-term results with weight loss you must remain active. You must be aware of your calorie intake. You must manage portion control. There are three major parameters that identify long-term weight loss success.

- Success on a weight maintenance program is defined as losing at least 10% of your current body weight and keeping it off for more than one year.

- Only 20% of people who lose weight are successful at maintaining the weight loss after one year.

- Once you maintain weight loss for 2-5 years, there is a greater chance that you'll have long-term success.

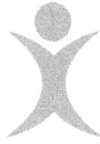

TIP

Encore Members Credit the Following Habits for Their Weight Loss Success

- Maintaining the healthy rituals learned during the first six weeks on the Encore program.

- Counting calories each day.

- Continuing to be mindful of journaling the food and drinks consumed.

- Daily journaling.

- Exercising or being in motion a minimum of 30 minutes per day, 5 days a week.

- Actively managing portion control.

- Avoiding all sweet drinks.

- Participating in nutritional coaching or group sessions at least twice per month.

ESSENTIALS OF THE ENCORE MAINTENANCE PROGRAM

Encore's 8-week maintenance program, Maintain for Life, includes:

- ➢ Physical Exam by an Encore Healthcare Provider or Video Conference Review of Medical Data

- ➢ Dietary Supplements & Vitamins

- ➢ Customized Meal Plan

- ➢ Wellness Coaching & Support

MAKING THE RIGHT CHOICES

Remember, to lose a pound of fat per week, you need to eliminate 3,500 calories from your weekly diet. That translates into consuming 500 fewer calories per day for seven (7) days. You should never eat simply because you are sad, happy, unhappy or angry. Instead of eating, vent your frustration with activity and movement. Vent your frustration by being mindful of your goal.

Maintenance and Weight Stabilization are achieved by being honest with yourself and by participating in activities that support your new lifestyle. Here are a few suggestions.

- Make sure your methods are sustainable.. Honestly, can you consistently get up every morning at 5 a.m. to work out? Perhaps exercising every other day, alternating cardio and weight lifting, is more realistic.

- Suggest business meetings be conducted in conference rooms or offices versus restaurants. Non-food meetings can be quite productive and focused.

- Don't feel pressured to declare that you're not eating dessert or drinking alcoholic beverages.

- Evaluate the health habits of your friends and close associates and determine if their habits are impacting you.

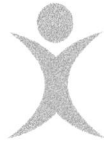

TIP

Continue to engage in exercise and
dietary rituals as a way of life...
you'll be happy you did!

Meal Planning

Our goal is to promote overall wellness. We firmly believe that there are many factors to keep in mind when meal planning. The size and composition of your food plate is an important factor.

We believe it is important to balance your plate and recommend the following suggestions:

- Fill ½ of the plate with non-starchy vegetables such as broccoli, carrots, cauliflower or green beans

- Fill ¼ of the plate with a starch, grain or starchy vegetable such as corn, peas or potatoes

- Use fat-free/low-fat milk or milk products

- Fill ¼ of the plate with lean meat, poultry or fish

If you choose a plant-based protein, such as dried beans, as your protein source, monitor the total caloric content to avoid adding hidden calories.

The actual number of calories each person needs to consume to avoid weight gain varies and depends on your body's metabolism. Consult with your Encore Healthcare Provider to determine your number.

Dietary Suggestions

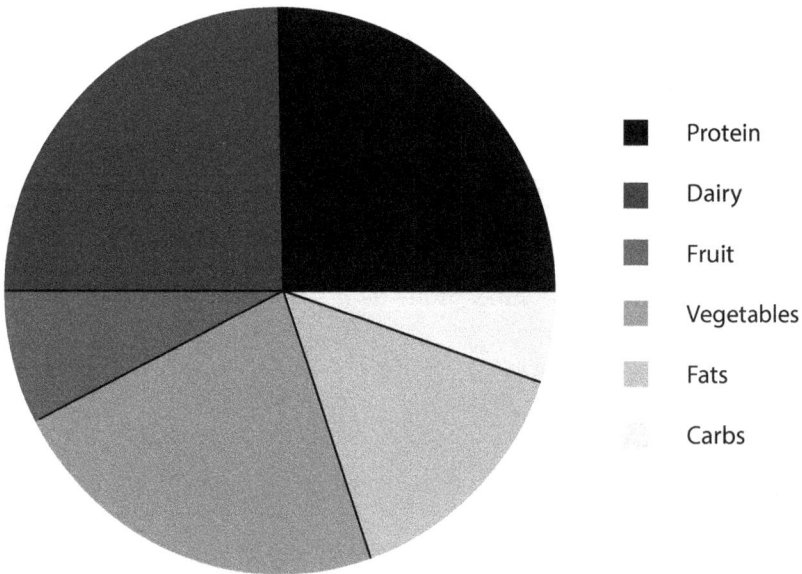

Legend:
- Protein
- Dairy
- Fruit
- Vegetables
- Fats
- Carbs

Eat a minimum of 3-4 cups of vegetables per day:

- Dark leafy greens are best.

- Swiss chard, spinach, collards, mustard and turnip greens, asparagus, cucumbers, broccoli, brussels sprouts, lettuce, celery, and carrots are also a favorite as they are high in Vitamin A

Select 2 servings of whole grain each day, with a minimum of 3 grams of fiber:

- Whole grains include oatmeal, buckwheat, whole wheat bread, quinoa, brown rice or Special K Protein Plus cereal.

Select a maximum of 2 tablespoons of heart-healthy fats and oils:

- Includes nuts, unsalted olives

- Natural peanut butter

- As a salad dressing alternative, try fresh salsa, lemon juice or balsamic vinegar & extra-virgin olive oil

PORTION CONTROL

As you plan meals, it's important to always practice portion control. Even if you eat healthy, it's possible to gain weight. If your portions are too large and exceed your calorie count for each meal, you will experience weight gain. As a general guideline, you can often estimate portion size by using the palm of your hand. Learning portion control requires that you always remain mindful of your goals. Over time, you can learn to recognize the appropriate amount of food you need to consume to feel satisfied. You can stay within your calorie count for the day and feel satisfied. During this process, you will find the correct portion size that works for you.

The goal is to set the stage for cultivating a healthy caloric environment. Achieving long-term weight management success requires continued focus and mindfulness of your goal at home, work and when dining out.

Maximize Your Weight Loss

It's important to acknowledge when you've met a goal or turned a corner. Reward yourself with something that is meaningful to you, something that makes you happy but that also supports your ultimate goal of managing your weight. Food should not be the reward!

The cornerstone to your long-term success is the continued use of the healthy rituals that lead to and maintain healthy habits. Dietary rituals and their related behaviors serve as the catalyst for your success. The following dietary rituals and related behaviors should be reviewed on a daily basis. Reinforce your use of these guidelines by reading them daily. Repetition of the correct process always paves the way to success. Use these rituals and behaviors as building blocks on your journey to healthy eating.

- Maintain the habit of selecting foods from a variety of groups.

- Consume balanced essential dietary nutrients to include proteins, fruits, vegetables and whole grains.

- Bake, grill or boil all meat and fish selections

- Eat boneless or skinless chicken and turkey cutlets. Eat lean ground turkey and lean beef cuts. Eat lentils, egg whites and cottage cheese.

- Clams and oysters are high in iron. Use them.

- Do not bread or deep-fry fish, seafood or vegetables. Select fat-free or skim milk.

- Select at least 2 servings of fruit each day.

- Eat more berries! Berries are loaded with antioxidants and contain less sugar than apples. During the fall and winter months you can substitute frozen berries.

- Low-sugar snacks include grapefruit, oranges, cantaloupe, raspberries, blackberries and blueberries and are typically available year-round. Use them as a main part of your diet.

- Practice portion control; when in doubt, no larger than the palm of your hand is generally a good portion-size measuring tool.

New habit formation and maintenance requires constant reinforcement. Rituals are the bricks that build new habits. Our behavior changes falters when we forget our rituals. Our memories are never really erased; they're just forgotten. Forgetting is similar to misfiling a document. If we rummage through the filing cabinet long enough we can find that lost document. That is, if we're looking in the correct cabinet. With the correct recall button we can restore our memories. All that is required to remember an event, a song, or a feeling is the correct stimulus that triggers the playback.

Similarly, you can use your daily rituals as stimuli to recall your healthy habits. Increase your willpower. Use the following daily rituals and social rituals as a platform for maintaining your health and weight loss success.

Daily Rituals

- Increase your level of physical activity to one hour per day, rather than 30 minutes, three to five times per week.

- Focus on a diet that is low in fat and high in low glycemic carbohydrates.

- Make sure your daily calorie intake from fat does not exceed 30%.

- Count your carbohydrates, keeping them below 60 grams per day.

- Eat breakfast daily and on a regular schedule.

- Enjoy a healthy salad with lunch and dinner.

- Monitor your weight daily and count the number of calories you're consuming.

- When you fall off your regimen, immediately adjust your caloric intake to get back on track.

SOCIAL RITUALS

- Surround yourself with inspiring and supportive family, co-workers and friends.

- Remind yourself daily how far you've come on this journey. You've invested time and emotions in your weight loss journey that you can never get back again. Why start over?

- Don't allow your social network to pressure you into eating poorly. What you see everyone ordering does not apply to you. Consider yourself the group health leader!

- Get in the habit of rewarding yourself with something you value other than food.

You have worked hard to achieve weight loss success. Weight maintenance within a healthy range is a key parameter that will determine the length of your life. Measurement and categorization of your weight history, blood pressure, blood sugar, cholesterol, lean body mass, physical activity and smoking history directly relate to how long and how healthy your life will be.

The following rituals should serve as guidelines for living a healthier and longer life.

To <u>Maintain and Stabilize</u> Your Weight:

- Water is the key to weight maintenance; you must continue to drink a minimum of 8 glasses per day (2-3 liters).

- Eating 5 small meals prevents overeating.

- Think of yourself as feeling full and satisfied.

- Stay focused on and mindful of your health goal.

- Maintain a consistent eating pattern across weekdays and weekends.

- Continue to avoid fried foods and fast foods.

- Embrace a sugar-free lifestyle; use Stevia, agave nectar or raw honey as sweeteners.

- Make one-slice sandwiches.

- Beware of empty, liquid calories.

- Season your food with herbs and spices; reduce salt intake.

- Prepare food without using cooking oils or butter; try a fat-free cooking spray or extra-virgin olive oil.

- To control fats and calories, prepare meals at home as often as possible.

- To aid in digestion, complete dinner at least 3½ hours before bedtime.

- Enjoy a low-calorie salad with lunch and dinner.

- Limit carbonated drinks.

- Before weighing, empty your bladder and bowel.

- Continue to weigh yourself daily, unclothed using the same scale.

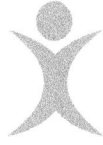

PHYSICAL ACTIVITY

The following are two great reasons to combine exercise with your current diet and nutrition program.

1. Exercise helps you burn fat and calories. Cardiovascular exercise or aerobic activity is among the best way to boost your body's metabolism and melt fat. A minimum of 20 to 30 minutes of aerobic exercise three to four times per week, like brisk walking, jogging or even dancing, will help you burn calories to slim down.

2. Exercise also helps you push through your plateau. For those who prefer to diet over working out, adding physical activity could shatter that ceiling that you can't seem to reach. Burning an extra 500 calories a day

will add to 3,500 calories a week, which is the number of calories that equals one pound lost (or gained). Doing the following activities for 30-60 minutes can help you burn those unwanted calories:

a. Salsa dancing

b. Running

c. Stair climbing

d. Cycling

Your workout program should include strength (resistance training), cardiovascular endurance (brisk walking, running, biking, elliptical) and flexibility (stretching) training. Each session should include a warm-up, the main workout, cool down and stretching.

The following section outlines the components of a complete fitness program and includes diagrams of several exercise routines. It also includes a helpful chart that illustrates the number of repetitions you'd complete to lose fat versus gain muscle.

FITNESS SUCCESS 101

GOAL:

1. Exercise your body 3-5 times per week for 30-60 minutes per session

   a. Resistance: 2-3 times/week

   b. Cardiovascular: 2 times/week

   c. Stretch daily

   d. Rest: 1-2 days/week

2. Commit to a resistance, cardiovascular and stretching program

3. Create a complementary fitness and nutrition program. (Remember that 3,500 calories equals 1 pound, which means that you have to burn or have a deficit of 3,500 calories to lose 1 pound.)

   a. For maximum results, a workout/ fitness program should be followed during and after any nutrition/weight loss program.

4. Track fitness and nutrition activities and program

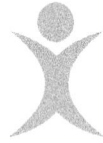

TIP

THREE COMPONENTS OF A COMPLETE EXERCISE PROGRAM:

- *Resistance*

- *Cardiovascular*

- *Stretching*

What is Resistance Exercise?

Any exercise using resistance tools such as dumbbells, machines, cables, tubing or balls to increase muscle endurance and strength, such as squats, shoulder press and push-ups.

Getting Started:

    a. Warm Up

    b. Do a Light Stretch

    c. Do 10-15 Reps of each Exercise / 3-4 sets preferably

    d. Cool Down

    e. Stretch

What is Cardiovascular Exercise?

Cardiovascular exercise is a form of exercise designed to work the cardiovascular system, improving lung and heart health along with improving the condition of the musculoskeletal system. The primary goal of cardiovascular exercise is to get the heart rate up and keep it up for a sustained period. Jogging, cycling and aerobics classes are some common examples of cardiovascular exercise.

Getting Started:

a. Warm Up

b. Do a Light Stretch

c. Cardio routine: 30-60 minutes

d. Cool Down

e. Stretch

Why Should I Stretch?

Stretching improves flexibility, which allows you to move your joints and muscles through their full range of motion. Flexibility is a key element of fitness; it can enhance physical performance, relieve muscle tension and stiffness and, most importantly, prevent injuries. You should stretch after a warm-up and/or when cooling down after a workout, since it is easier and safer to stretch a warm muscle than a cold one. Warm-ups bring blood to the muscles and make injuries from stretching less likely.

Combined Program:

    a. Warm Up (5-10 minutes of light cardio)

    b. Light Stretch

    c. Resistance Exercise: 30-60 minutes

    d. Cardio Routine: 30 minutes

    e. Cool Down

    f. Stretch

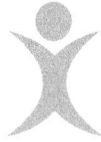

TIP

ESTABLISH YOUR GOAL

Someone who is trying to gain muscle should eat and train differently from someone who is trying to lose weight.

TRAIN FOR YOUR GOAL					
GOAL	EXERCISE	WEIGHT	SET	REPS	REST
Fat Loss	Varies	Light to Moderate	1 to 3	12-16 reps	0-30 sec.
Muscle Gain	Varies	Heavy	3 to 6	6-8 reps	2-5 min.
Weight Gain	Varies	Heavy	3 to 6	6-8 reps	2-5 min.
Maintain/ Optimal Health	Varies	Light to Moderate	1 to 3	10-12 reps	30-60 sec.

Your fitness routine should include exercises for the following muscle groups:

1. Deltoids (shoulders) – Try lateral extensions, shoulder press

2. Biceps – Try bicep curls

3. Triceps – Try triceps extensions

4. Chest – Try push-ups or bench press

5. Back – Try pull-ups, lat pull downs, flys

6. Abs/Core – Try bicycles, plank holds

7. Quadriceps – Try lunges

8. Hamstrings/gluteus maximus – Try squats

9. Calves – Try calf raises

There are approximately 260 muscles in the body, so why work on only seven muscles, and why these seven? Well, it's all about getting the most bang for your effort. When exercising, it's best to work on your large muscle groups. It's as if you are fine-tuning a regular car engine as opposed to an engine in a toy boat. The larger the muscle, the more metabolic benefit you receive, and the bigger the payoff when it comes to weight maintenance.

The Simple 7 group consists of the fewest number of muscle groups one has to work on to achieve maximum benefit in an exercise routine. You can exercise more or fewer muscle groups, but if you attack these particular muscles, then you will achieve maximum benefit. Also, it's important to realize that the body is a balanced machine, and you must work the lower with the upper, and the back with the front. The seven muscle groups provide total balance in an easy way.

Sample Exercises

Use the "Goal-based Sets, Reps and Rest" chart on page 92 to determine your appropriate program. If using weights, adjust them so you can complete each repetition. It shouldn't be easy, you should struggle to complete each repetition, but it shouldn't be so difficult that you cannot complete the set.

SQUAT

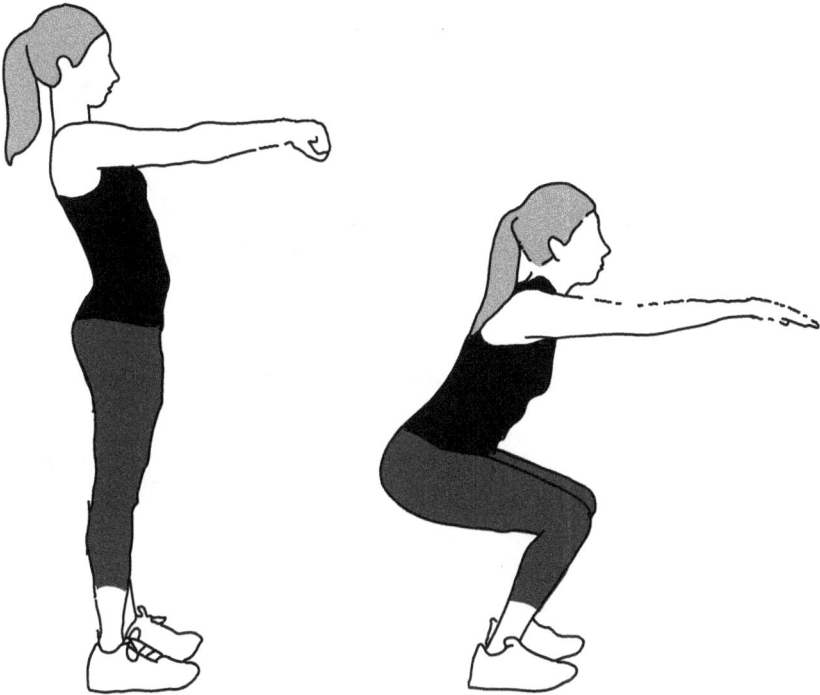

1. Stand straight with feet hip-width apart.
   Your feet should be directly under your
   hips. Place your hands in front of you.

2. Stand up tall, put your shoulders back, lift
   your chest, pull in your abdominal muscles
   and tighten your stomach muscles.

3. Lower yourself down, as if sitting on a chair
   or bench. Bend your knees while keeping
   your upper body as straight as possible, as
   if you were lowering yourself onto a seat

behind you. Lower yourself as far as you can without leaning your upper body more than a few inches forward. Your upper body should be perpendicular to the floor, and your thighs should be parallel to the floor.

Tip: Don't allow your knees to go too far forward. You don't want them to extend past your toes.

4. Be careful not to lock your knees when you reach a standing position.

PUSH-UP

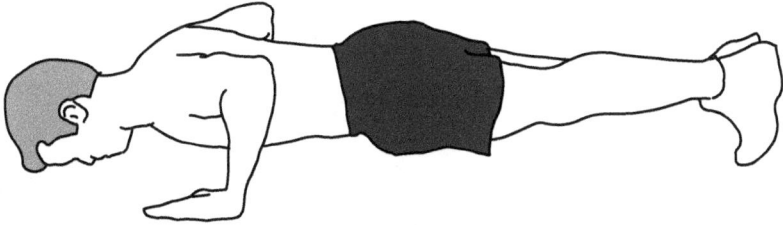

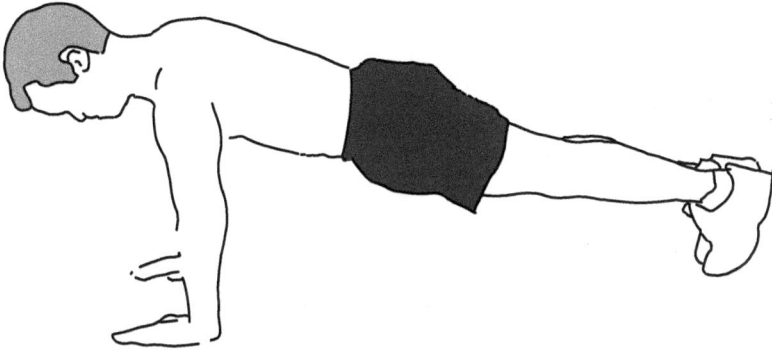

1. Lie down on your stomach; place your hands slightly more than shoulder-width apart. Tuck your toes under your feet to support your body. Tighten your abdominal muscles, keep your back in one straight line and exhale as you push yourself off the floor.

2. Once your arms are straight, inhale as you lower yourself to the floor; stop when your elbows reach a 90-degree bend. Keep your body from touching the floor.

3. Exhale and push yourself away from the floor. Don't lock your elbows, and don't bend your back.

4. Repeat steps 1-3.

PUSH-UP ON KNEES

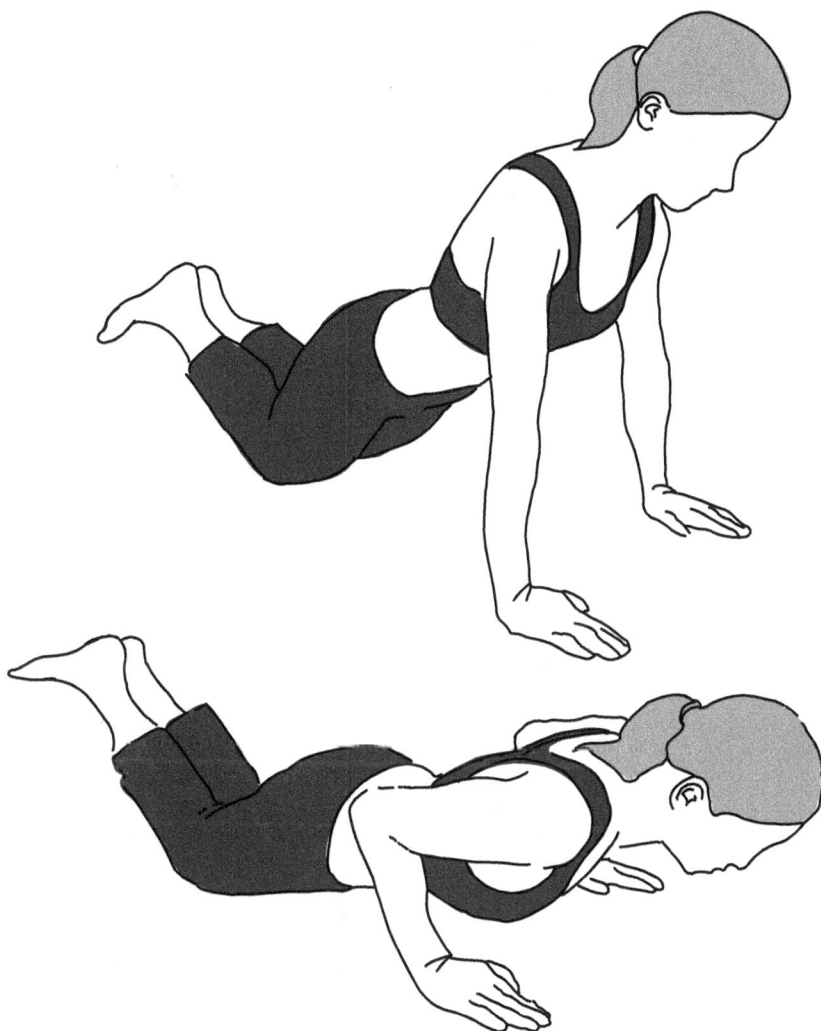

1. Place your hands and knees on the floor. Keeping your gluteus and abs tight, your back should be in one diagonal line with your head and neck, and your feet should be lifted from the floor.

2. Inhale as you lower yourself to the floor, stopping as your elbows reach a 90-degree bend. Keep your body from touching the floor.

3. Exhale and push yourself away from the floor. Don't lock your elbows, and don't bend your back.

4. Repeat steps 1-3.

SEATED LAT PULL DOWNS

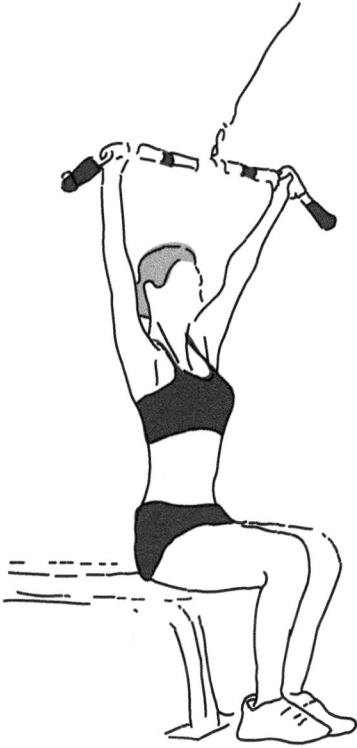

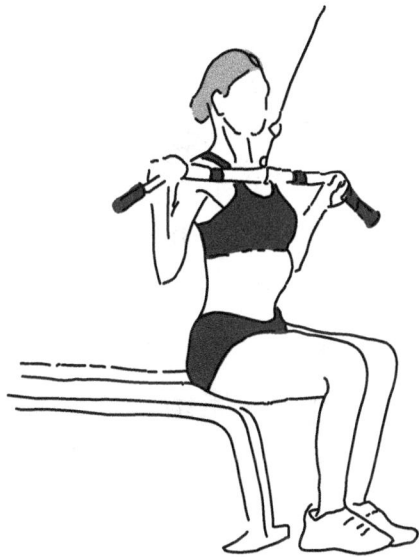

1. Sit in the machine and anchor your body by securing your thighs under the pad.

2. Brace your core and abdominal muscles to stabilize the spine. Grasp the bar with your hands wider than shoulder-width apart, palms facing forward and thumbs wrapped around the bar.

3. With your elbows straight overhead, pull your shoulder blades down and back. Do not allow your back to arch. Lean back slightly. Keep your feet firmly on the floor and your head aligned with your spine. Maintain these engagements throughout the exercise.

4. Exhale as you pull the bar to the top or mid-section of your chest while lowering your shoulder blades. Pull the bar in a motion that brings your elbows toward the sides of your torso, driving your elbows toward the floor. Do not lean back any farther as you pull the bar down.

5. Pause briefly. In a slow and controlled manner, straighten your elbows and return the bar to starting position without locking your elbows, allowing your shoulder blades to rise slightly.

6. Repeat steps 1-5.

SEATED SHOULDER PRESS

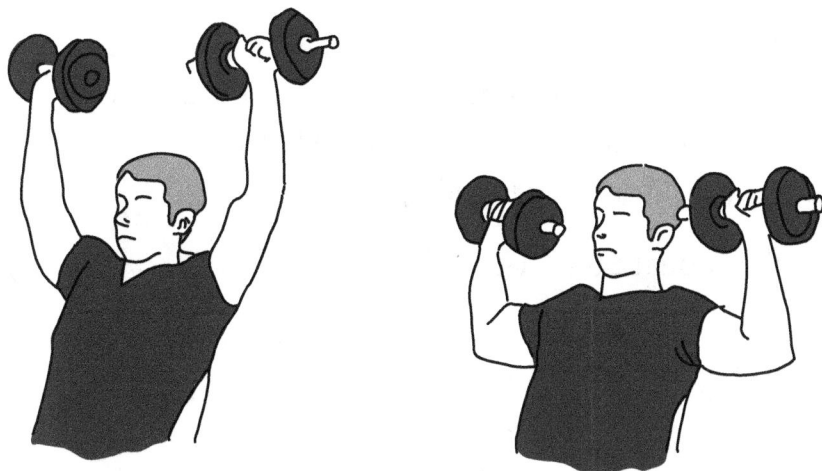

1. While holding a dumbbell in each hand, sit on a military press bench or utility bench that has back support. Place the dumbbells upright on top of your thighs.

2. Now raise the dumbbells to shoulder height one at a time using your thighs to help propel them up into position.

3. Make sure to rotate your wrists so that the palms of your hands are facing forward. Make sure your shoulders are at a 90-degree angle on each side. This is your starting position. Brace your abdominals and keep your lower back against the bench at all times.

4. Now, exhale and push the dumbbells upward until they touch at the top.

5. Then, after a brief pause at the top contracted position, inhale as you slowly lower the weights back down to the starting position while inhaling.

6. Repeat Steps 1-5.

PLANKS

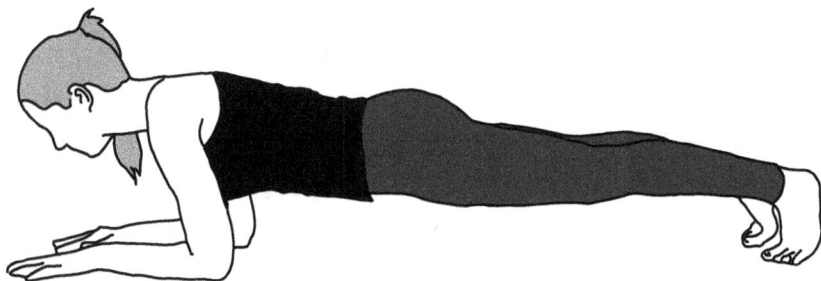

1. Lie face down on a mat, resting on your forearms, palms flat on the floor and your elbows directly underneath your shoulders.

2. Push off the floor, raising up onto your toes and resting on your elbows.

3. Keep your back flat, in a straight line from head to heels.

4. Tilt your pelvis and contract your abdominals to prevent your rear end from sticking up in the air or sagging in the middle.

5. Hold for 20 to 60 seconds and lower.

   Tip: You can keep your knees on the ground to take the pressure off your back or to modify the movement.

WEIGHT, SETS, REPS AND REST

HOW MANY REPS/SETS TO DO?

Your decision should be based on your goals. In general:

- For fat loss: 1-3 sets of 10-12 reps using enough weight that you can ONLY complete the desired reps.

- To gain muscle: 3-6 sets of 6-8 reps to fatigue. For beginners, give yourself several weeks of conditioning before going to this level. You may need a spotter for many exercises.

- For health and endurance: 1-3 sets of 12-16 reps using enough weight that you can ONLY complete the desired reps.

HOW LONG TO REST BETWEEN EXERCISES/WORKOUT SESSIONS?

This will depend on your goal as well. Higher intensity exercise (i.e., when lifting heavy weights) and muscle gain workouts require a longer rest. When lifting to fatigue, it takes an average of 2 to 5 minutes for your muscles to rest for the next set. When using lighter weight and more repetitions (fat loss or endurance), it takes between 30 seconds and 1 minute for your muscles to rest.

How Often Should I Train Each Muscle Group?

The American College of Sports Medicine recommends training each muscle group 2 to 3 times a week. But, the number of times you lift each week will depend on your training method. In order for muscles to repair and grow, you'll need about 48 hours of rest between workout sessions. If you're training at a high intensity, take a longer rest.

Recommendation: Work out 3-5 days/week.

- 3 days/week: Resistance training 1 day and cardio 2 days
- 4 days/week: Resistance training 2 days and cardio 2 days
- 5 days/week: Resistance training 2 days and cardio 3 days

How Much Weight to Lift?

Choosing how much weight to lift is often based on how many reps and sets you're doing. The general rule is to lift enough weight that you can ONLY complete the desired number of reps. In other words, you want to work to fatigue. However, if you're a beginner or if you have medical or health conditions, you may need to avoid complete fatigue and just find a weight that challenges you at a level you can handle.

How do you know how much weight you need to challenge your body? Here are a few tips to help you decide:

- The larger muscles of the glutes, thighs, chest and back can usually handle heavier weight than the smaller muscles of the shoulders, arms, abs and calves.

- You'll usually lift more weight on a machine than with dumbbells. With machines, you're using both arms and/or legs to complete the exercise, while with dumbbells, each limb works. independently. So, if you can handle 30 or 40 pounds on a chest press machine, you may only be able to handle 15 or 20 pounds with dumbbells.

- If you're a beginner, it's more important to focus on good form than lifting heavy weights.

- It may take several workouts to figure out how much weight you need.

The easiest way to determine how much weight to use on each lift is to start with lower weights.

1. Pick up a light weight and do a warm-up set of the exercise of your choice, aiming for about 10-16 reps.

2. For set 2, increase your weight by 5 or more pounds and perform your goal number of repetitions. If you can do more than your desired number of reps, choose a heavier weight for your 3rd set.

3. In general, you should be lifting enough weight that you can ONLY do the desired reps. Expect to struggle by the last rep but still be able to finish in good form.

GOAL-BASED SETS, REPS AND REST

FAT LOSS					
EXERCISE	VARIATION	WEIGHT	SET	REPS	REST
Squat		Light to Moderate	1 to 3	12-16 reps	0-30 sec.
Push-up		Light to Moderate	1 to 3	12-16 reps	0-30 sec.
Lat Pull Downs		Light to Moderate	1 to 3	12-16 reps	0-30 sec.
Shoulder Press		Light to Moderate	1 to 3	12-16 reps	0-30 sec.
Planks		Light to Moderate	1 to 3	30-60 sec.	0-30 sec.

MUSCLE GAIN (HYPERTROPHY)					
EXERCISE	VARIATION	WEIGHT	SET	REPS	REST
Squat		Heavy	3 to 6	6-8 reps	2-5 min.
Push-up		Heavy	3 to 6	6-8 reps	2-5 min.
Lat Pull Downs		Heavy	3 to 6	6-8 reps	2-5 min.
Shoulder Press		Heavy	3 to 6	6-8 reps	2-5 min.
Planks		Heavy	3 to 6	30-60 seconds	2-5 min.

HEALTH AND ENDURANCE					
EXERCISE	VARIATION	WEIGHT	SET	REPS	REST
Squat		Light to Moderate	1 to 3	10-12 reps	30-60 sec.
Push-up		Light to Moderate	1 to 3	10-12 reps	30-60 sec.
Lat Pull Downs		Light to Moderate	1 to 3	10-12 reps	30-60 sec.
Shoulder Press		Light to Moderate	1 to 3	10-12 reps	30-60 sec.
Planks		Light to Moderate	1 to 3	30-60 seconds	30-60 sec.

Gym Shy?

Try this program if you prefer to stay out of the gym. Need: Small weights, mat, exercise ball.

Our challenging total body workouts can be performed two to three times each week to improve your core, your total body strength and your cardiovascular endurance. Maintain great form while performing each exercise with minimal rest until you complete each combination. Then rest for one minute. You can either repeat the same combination if you want to challenge yourself or you can move on to the next combination listed in the series. Remember, challenge yourself and don't give up!

SAMPLE 7-DAY AT-HOME TRAINING SCHEDULE

The following is a brief example of what your workouts may look like for the week.

MONDAY:	Perform Series #1
TUESDAY:	Rest day
WEDNESDAY:	Perform Series #2
THURSDAY:	Rest day
FRIDAY:	Cardiovascular activity of your choice or perform Series #1 again if you want to challenge yourself.
SATURDAY:	Cardiovascular activity of your choice for at least 30 minutes or attend a yoga class.
SUNDAY:	Rest day

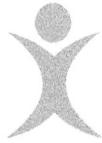

TIP

THINGS TO REMEMBER

1. Warm up for at least 5-8 minutes before each workout to get your heart rate pumping and to prevent injuries. Example: Light jog or walking in place.

2. Perform light stretches for 2-3 minutes after your warm-up. Example: Shoulder roll forward and back and neck stretch.

3. Stay hydrated: Have your water bottle handy.

STRENGTH AND CONDITIONING SERIES #1

Stationary lunge (10-12 reps)
Bicep curl (10-12 reps)
Jumping jacks for 60 seconds
Basic squat (10-12 reps)
Plank hold for 30 seconds
Jumping jacks for 60 seconds
Dumbbell chest fly on stability ball (10 reps)
Alternating side lunge with a thrust (5 each side)

Repeat this combination twice to challenge yourself.

Strength and Conditioning Series #2

Dumbbell row (8-10 each side)
Side lunges (10 each side); no weights
Dumbbell chest fly on stability ball (16-20)
60 seconds simulated jump rope
Vertical leg crunch (lying on back, both legs straight up in the air, both hands behind your head, crunch) (16-20)
40 mountain climbers
Military shoulder press (10-12)
Plank hold for 60 seconds

Repeat this combination twice to challenge yourself!

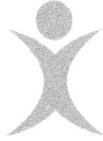

We are confident that once you establish the program cycle that works for you, and you start to see and feel the fruits of your labor, you will be more than happy that you took this journey.

Join the Encore movement and share your journey with us. Simply visit our website to contact us and tell us your story. Encore membership can change your life and the life of your family.

www.encoreweightloss.com

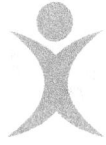

REFERENCE TOOLS

The following section provides tools and resources to help you on your journey.

CALORIE CONTENT – FRUITS & VEGETABLES

FRUIT CALORIES AND MACRO-NUTRIENTS

Fruit	Serving	Calories	Carbs (g)	Protein (g)	Fat (g)
Apple	raw, with skin, 100 g = 1 small	52	13.8	0.3	0.2
Apricot	raw, with skin, 100 g = 3 apricots	48	11.1	1.0	0.4
Avocado	raw, no skin, 100 g	160	8.5	2.0	
Banana	1 medium	94	21.7	1.1	0.3
Boysenberries	raw, 1 cup	75	18.4	1.0	0.6
Blueberries	raw, 1 cup	81	20.5	1.7	0.6
Dates	1 cup, pitted, chopped	490	130.8	3.6	0.7
Grapefruit	1 medium	82	20.5	1.5	0.3
Grapes	1 cup, seedless, red or green	114	28.3	1.0	1.0
Kiwi	1 medium, 2.7 oz, no skin	46	11.2	0.8	0.3
Lemon	1 medium, 2 oz	17	5.4	0.6	0.2
Melon	cantaloupe, 1 medium wedge, 2.4 oz	24	5.7	0.6	0.2
Nectarine	1 medium	67	15.9	1.2	0.5
Oranges	1 large, 6.5 oz	86	21.5	1.7	0.2
Peaches	1 medium, 3.5 oz	42	10.8	0.7	0.0
Pear	1 medium, 5.8 oz	98	25.1	0.7	0.7
Pineapple	1 cup, diced, 5.5 oz	76	19.2	0.6	0.6
Plums	1 medium, 2.3 oz	36	8.6	0.5	0.4
Raspberries	1 cup, 4.3 oz	60	14.1	1.2	0.6
Strawberries	1 cup, halves, 5.4 oz	46	10.6	0.9	0.5
Watermelon	1 wedge, 10 oz	92	20.6	1.7	1.1

VEGETABLE CALORIES AND MACRO-NUTRIENTS

Fruit	Serving	Calories	Carbs (g)	Protein (g)	Fat (g)
Asparagus	raw, 4 medium spears, 2 oz	11	2.2	1.3	0.1
Beans, Kidney	boiled, 1/2 cup, 3 oz	108	19.4	7.2	0.4
Broccoli	1 cup chopped, 3 oz	35	5.6	2.4	0.3
Cabbage	1 cup shredded, 5 oz	41	9.8	2.1	0.1
Carrots	1 cup chopped	52	12.3	1.3	0.3
Cauliflower	1 cup chopped, 3.5 oz	23	4.1	1.8	0.4
Celery	1 cup chopped, 3.5 oz	14	3.6	0.7	0.2
Corn (kernels)	1/2 cup kernels, 3.5 oz	354	82.3	10.8	4.3
Corn on cob	1 large ear, 5.5 oz	140	33.3	4.7	1.1
Cucumber	1/2 cup slices (with skin), 2 oz	7	1.3	0.3	0.1
Lentils	1/2 cup boiled, 3.5 oz	115	19.9	8.9	0.4
Lettuce (iceberg)	1 cup shredded, 1.9 oz	8	1.7	0.5	0.1
Mushrooms	1/2 cup pieces, 2.5 oz	20	3.8	1.4	0.4
Onion	1/2 cup chopped, 3 oz	36	8.6	0.8	0.1
Peas	1/4 cup, 1.5 oz	36	6.7	2.3	0.1
Peppers (bell or sweet)	1 cup sliced, 3.2 oz	18	4.2	0.8	0.2
Potatoes	1 potato, baked with skin, 7 oz	255	58.1	7.0	0.4
Pumpkin	1/2 cup mashed, 4 oz	23	5.6	0.8	0.1
Spinach	1/2 cup, 3 oz	20	3.2	2.6	0.3
Sweet potato	1 cup, baked, with skin, 7 oz	180	41.4	4.0	0.4
Tomato	1 tomato, raw, 2.2 oz	11	2.4	0.6	0.1

RE-STOCKING YOUR KITCHEN

As you stock your kitchen, consider the following fiber-rich foods and drinks, which are known to help you feel full and satisfied:

WATER is the least expensive, simplest way to curb appetite and keep your body functioning properly. Add slices of lemon, lime, cucumber, fresh ginger or a few drops of juice to flavor. Dehydration slows down your metabolism, so keep hydrated throughout the day.

GREEK YOGURT has twice the protein of regular yogurt – some brands contain more than 20 grams of protein per serving. Choose low-fat, plain varieties and add fresh fruit, if desired.

EGGS are inexpensive. egg protein sticks with you and can be eaten with any meal. If you're watching your cholesterol, use half egg whites in the mix.

WHOLE GRAIN BREADS AND PRODUCTS digest slower than white flour products. Read the label to make sure the first ingredient listed is a whole grain, such as wheat or oats. You'll also find whole grains in crackers, pasta and cereal.

SKIM MILK can help curb your appetite. Try a glass of fat-free milk, which contains about 9 grams of protein and 300 mg OF CALCIUM. Many people get less than half their daily calcium requirement.

CHEESE with 6 or more grams of protein per 1-ounce serving. Cheese is a perfect snack with a few whole grain crackers or an apple. Choose a low-fat cheese such as mozzarella, Babybel OR Laughing Cow. You will be satisfied with a small piece.

PROTEIN-PLUS WHOLE GRAIN CEREAL can be a healthy snack any time. Choose wisely. Look for whole grains as the first ingredient and look for brands without added carbohydrates (sugar, corn syrup or fructose) listed in the first few ingredients.

LEAN POULTRY is a great way to get lean protein, but control portion size. No more than 3 oz per serving size.

BERRIES: You may know that strawberries are high in fiber, but did you know that raspberries actually have EVEN more FIBER?

- Raspberries have about 8 grams of fiber per cup

- Strawberries have about 3 grams
- Blueberries are another good high-fiber choice
- All berries contain disease-fighting antioxidants

CHICKPEAS are versatile; you can make hummus to use as a dip or sandwich spread. Add them to soups and stews or toss them on salads and pasta dishes. One half-cup of roasted chickpeas has 100 calories, 5 grams of protein and 4 grams of fiber.

For a savory snack, roast chickpeas for 30 or 40 minutes at 425 degrees until crispy. toss with salt, pepper and/or Cajun spices.

GREEN TEA: studies suggest that drinking 2-4 cups of green tea daily will help burn calories. Consider replacing high-calorie drinks with green tea, WHICH CONTAINS NO CALORIES.

TURNIPS OR RUTABAGAS: these root veggies can be diced and roasted, added to stews or boiled and mashed as a substitute for white potatoes.

- Contain about 5 grams of fiber per cup.

Tip: Don't discard those vitamin-rich leafy tops – you can sauté them as you would spinach and other green LEAFY VEGETABLEs.

BLACK BEANS can provide protein without fat. Reduce your fat consumption by making black bean burgers: Drain a can of black beans and mash; add garlic and onion powder to taste; mix with one egg white to hold together. Form into patties and sauté. Add a slice of pepper jack cheese to boost the flavor.

PEARS are a high-fiber, low calorie snack, and they contain twice as much fiber as apples:

Slice into salads, roast alongside pork tenderloin or bake whole for dessert. If you don't like softer types of pears, such as Bartlett, try firmer varieties, such as Bosc.

OKRA is a great source of soluble fiber. Soluble fiber helps keep you full and lowers cholesterol. Add OKRA TO soup or gumbo as a natural thickener. Okra pairs especially well with tomatoes, chickpeas and feta cheese for a vegetarian stew. You'll find it in the frozen foods aisle.

LENTILS are nutritional powerhouses, containing 9 grams of protein and 8 grams of fiber per half-cup serving, which is more than many other legumes. They cook fast (in about 20 minutes). Lentils come in many different types and go well in soups or as a quick side dish.

LEAN BEEF can be part of a sensible diet because it's protein-rich (3 ounces of some cuts contains more than 30 grams of protein). Look for leaner cuts with less fatty marbling, such as tenderloin, roast or 98% lean ground beef.

BROWN RICE: like whole wheat bread, brown rice contains more nutrients than the white variety. Plus, it has 3 to 4 times the fiber. Brown rice typically takes longer to cook, but you can now find pre-cooked brown rice to heat in the microwave or on the stove.

WHITE BEANS, such as cannellini or Great Northern, can be used as an alternative to kidney or black beans in soups and chili.

6 grams of protein and 6 grams of fiber, white beans stick with you and make you feel full longer.

GREENS are a great source of vitamins A

and C. Greens are high in minerals such as potassium and magnesium.

- Kale, spinach, Swiss chard and col-lard greens are rich in water, and keep you feeling full longer.
- Sauté fresh greens in low-sodium vegetable or chicken broth, add a drizzle of heart-healthy olive oil and a dash of red pepper. Top with crumbled feta cheese.

SUPER SEVEN Rx FOR WEIGHT LOSS

1. CHROMIUM

   Chromium is a mineral found in certain foods. The body needs only trace amounts of chromium, and deficiency of this mineral in humans is rare.

   Chromium picolinate works together with insulin produced by the pancreas to metabolize carbohydrates.

   Chromium picolinate has been used in alternative medicine as an aid to lowering cholesterol or improving the body's use of glucose (sugar). It is also commonly touted as a weight-loss supplement that aids in reducing body fat and increasing lean muscle. Not all uses for chromium picolinate have been approved by the FDA. Chromium picolinate should not be substituted for prescription medications.

   Chromium picolinate is often sold as an herbal supplement. There are no regulated manufacturing standards in place for many herbal compounds and some marketed supplements have been found to be contaminated with toxic metals or other drugs. Herbal/health supplements should be purchased from a reliable source to minimize the risk of contamination.

   Chromium picolinate may also be used for other purposes not listed in the chromium picolinate guide. Use chromium picolinate as directed on the label, or as your doctor has prescribed. Do not use this product in larger amounts or for longer than recommended.

Your healthcare provider may occasionally change your dose to make sure you get the best results from chromium picolinate. The recommended dietary allowance of chromium increases with age. Follow your healthcare provider's instructions. Your dose needs may change if you have an injury, illness or infection, if you are pregnant, if you are under stress or if you exercise more than usual.

Chromium picolinate is only part of a complete program of treatment that may also include diet, exercise and weight control. Follow your diet, medication and exercise routines very closely.

Tell your healthcare provider about all other medications you use, especially insulin or diabetes medications you take by mouth, steroid medications, nicotinic acid, stomach acid reducers, asthma or blood pressure medications, aspirin or NSAIDs (non-steroidal anti-inflammatory drugs).

2. CONJUGATED LINOLEIC ACID (CLA)
    Description: CLA is a varied form of the essential fatty acid linoleic acid. It is found in the red meat of cattle that are fed natural grasses. It is also found in eggs, poultry and safflower and corn oil. CLA is

mainly used as a supplement to reduce body fat. Animal and test tube studies have demonstrated its anticancer properties, but these results have yet to be proven in human studies.

Indications: Cancer prevention, weight loss.

Precautions: There are occasional reports of digestive upset.

Dosage: Take 1,000 mg two to three times daily.

3.   5-HYDROXYTRYPTOPHAN
Description: The supplement 5-HTP is an amino acid-like substance used as a precursor to make the neurotransmitter serotonin. Serotonin is important for balanced mood, sleep, pain control and other important functions of the body. This supplement is extracted from the seeds of the African plant Griffonia simplicifolia.

Indications: Anxiety, depression, fibromyalgia, food cravings (carbohydrates), insomnia, migraine headaches, seasonal affective disorder and weight loss.

Precautions: Large amounts may cause digestive upset, headaches or sleepiness. It should not be taken in conjunction with pharmaceutical antidepressant, anianxiety or other psychiatric medications.

Dosage: Take 50 to 100 mg three times daily on an empty stomach.

4. PYRUVATE

Pyruvate is the end product of glycolysis, which is converted into acetyl CoA that enters the Krebs cycle when there is sufficient oxygen available. When the oxygen is insufficient, **pyruvate** is broken down anaerobically, creating lactate in animals (including humans) and ethanol in plants.

5. L-CARNITINE

Function: energy production, heart function, triglyceride metabolism

Sources: Meat, dairy products

Optimal Intake: 250 to 500 mg

Deficiency Signs: Loss of muscle tone, recurrent infections, brain swelling, heart irregularities, high triglycerides, fatigue and failure to thrive

Toxicity: None

6. GREEN TEA

Description: This tea or supplemental extract is derived from the leaves of Camellia sinensis, the same plant that is used to make white and black tea. The leaves are lightly steamed and processed less than those of black tea, which accounts for green tea's high antioxidant properties. It has been found to contain very potent antioxidant activity, and it improves detoxification. Green tea is commonly available in liquid, tablet and capsule form.

Indications: Cancer, Cardiovascular disease, detoxification, digestive health and gingivitis.

Dosage: Take 100 to 200 mcg two to three times daily.

7.   ESSENTIAL FATTY ACIDS

FISH OIL

Description: Fish oil is the richest source of the omega-3 fatty acids DHA (docosahexaenoic acid) and EPA (eicosapentaenoic acid). Both DHA and EPA have antiflammatory effects. DHA plays an important role in brain function and joint health. EPA regulates inflammation, the immune system, blood clotting and circulation.

Indications: Arthritis, asthma, attention deficit disorder, bipolar disorder, cancer, cardiovascular disease, chronic obstructive pulmonary disease, depression, diabetes, high blood pressure, high cholesterol and triglycerides, inflammatory bowel disease, lupus, osteoporosis, preeclampsia, pregnancy, schizophrenia.

Precautions: Digestive upset (especially reflux and burping) may occur if fish oil product is not enteric-coated. Fish oil has a mild blood-thinning effect. Some people may have a rise in LDL cholesterol. This can be prevented with garlic supplementation.

Dosage: Take 3 to 5 grams total of EPA and DHA together for therapeutic purposes. Otherwise, take 1 to 2 grams total EPA and DHA together for preventative purposes.

FLAXSEED OIL
Description: Flaxseed oil is a rich source of alpha linolenic acid, an omega-3 fatty acid. Alpha linolenic acid is converted into DHA (docosahexaenoic acid) and EPA (eicosapentaenoic acid). It is used to reduce inflammation; promote healthy circulation and healthy skin, hair and nails; as well as to improve constipation. However, it has not been as well studied as fish oil has.

Indications: Arthritis, asthma, attention deficit disorder, bipolar disorder, cancer, cardiovascular disease, chronic obstructive pulmonary disease, constipation, depression, diabetes, high blood pressure, high cholesterol and triglycerides, inflammatory bowel diease and lupus.

Precautions: Too much flaxseed oil can cause diarrhea. Men with prostate cancer should avoid supplementation with flaxseed oil and use ground seeds instead. Flaxseed oil has a mild blood-thinning effect, so consult with your doctor before supplementation if you are on blood-thinning medication.

Dosage: Take 1 to 2 tablespoons or 8 to 12 capsules daily.

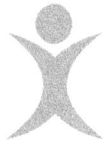

JOURNALING
TRACKING YOUR PROGRESS

TECHNOLOGIES

With the popularity of smart phones and apps solving everyday problems in the most resourceful of ways, creating meals on the fly has gotten easier right at our fingertips. Now, thanks to a bevy of food loving apps, meal planning has taken a new direction.

Apps make it easy with suggestions of what to cook, how to shop for it and where to keep track of all of those suggestions. All on cross-platform devices that sync between your desktop and mobile devices, making the pen-and-paper shopping list a thing of the past.

The popularity of applications and their usefulness depends upon your device and your perspective. The rating of applications for meal planning changes from time to time, so it's best to periodically research the best tools for you.

You'll find that various applications will serve as an example of how you can manage the information needed to successfully complete your health journey. The use of applications to record your caloric intake and gratitude journaling allows for rapid and complete sharing.

Sharing health data with your Encore Health Professional allows for a more successful health journey. It will give you an opportunity to receive useful feedback for continued success.

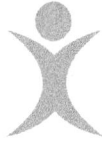

TIP

JOURNALING FOR SUCCESS

Medical studies clearly confirm that if you keep a journal of your dietary intake and gratitude, your chances for weight loss success are exponentially increased.

The following pages provide a template you can use to track this information and measure your progress.

DAILY JOURNAL

DATE: _____

BREAKFAST
TIME:

MEAL:

SNACK
TIME:

MEAL:

LUNCH
TIME:

MEAL:

SNACK
TIME:

MEAL:

DINNER
TIME:

MEAL:

EXERCISE:
TIME:

TYPES AND DURATION:

WEIGHT:
TIME:

1. *Today I am grateful for* _____

2. *Today I am grateful for* _____

3. *Today I am grateful for* _____

4. *Today I am grateful for* _____

5. *Today I am grateful for* _____

BIBLIOGRAPHY

1. Jensen MD, Ryan DH, Apocian CM, et al, 2013 AHA/ACC/TOS guidline for the management of overweight and obesity in adults: a report of the American College of Cardiology/American Heart Association Tas Force on Practive Guidlines and The Obesity Society. Circulation 2014; 129:S102.

2. Diabetes Prevention Program Research Group, Knowler WC, Fowler SE, et al, 10-year follow-up of diabetes incidence and weight loss in the Diabetes Prevention Program Outcomes Study. Lancet 2009; 374:1677.

3. Horvath K, Jeitler K, Siering U, et al. Long-term effects of weight-reducing interventions in hypertensive patients; systematic review and meta-analysis. Arch Intern Med 2008; 168:571

4. Douketis JD, Macie C, Thabane L, Williamson DF, Systematic review of long-term weight loss studies in obese adults: clinical significance and applicability to clinical practice. Int. J Oves (Lond) 2005; 29:1153

5. Poobalan AS, Aucott LS, Smith WC, et al. Long-term weight loss effects on all cause mortality in overweight/obese populations. Obes Rev 2007; 8:503

6. Sjostrom L. Review of the key results from the Swedish Ovese Subjects (sos) trial - a prospective controlled intervention study of bariatric surgery. J Intern Med 2013; 273:219

7. Leibel RL, Rosenbaum M, Hirsch J. Changes in energy expenditure resulting from altered body weight. N Engl J Med 1995; 332:621

8. Maynard LM, Serdula MK, Galuska DA, et al. Secular trends in desired weight of adults. Int J Obes (Lond) 2006; 30:1375

9. Leblanc ES, O'Connor E, Whitlock EP, et al. Effectiveness of primary care-relevant treatments for obesity in adults: a systematic evidence review for the U. S. Preventive Services Task Force. Ann Intern Med 2011; 155:434

10. Perri MG, Nezu AM, McKelvey WF, et al. Relapse precention training and problem solving therapy in the long-term management of obesity. J Consult Clin Psychol 2001; 69:722

11. Gloy VL, Briel M, Bhatt DL, et al. Bariatric surgery versus non-surgical treatment for obesity: a systematic review and meta-analysis of randomised controlled trials. BMJ 2013; 347:15934

NOTES

www.ingramcontent.com/pod-product-compliance
Lightning Source LLC
Chambersburg PA
CBHW060906280326
41934CB00007B/1213